Rafaela Julia Batista Veronezi

Spinal trauma in Goiânia/GO

Rafaela Julia Batista Veronezi

Spinal trauma in Goiânia/GO

Epidemiological study

ScienciaScripts

Imprint

Cover image: www.ingimage.com

This book is a translation from the original published under ISBN 978-613-9-70008-0.

Publisher:
Sciencia Scripts
is a trademark of
Dodo Books Indian Ocean Ltd. and OmniScriptum S.R.L publishing group

120 High Road, East Finchley, London, N2 9ED, United Kingdom
Str. Armeneasca 28/1, office 1, Chisinau MD-2012, Republic of Moldova, Europe
Printed at: see last page
ISBN: 978-620-8-15040-2

To my sons **Miguel** and **Moisés,** the protagonists of everything.

A love that never divides, always multiplies...

SUMMARY

CHAPTER 1

INTRODUCTION

Trauma is one of the main public health problems in all countries, regardless of socio-economic development. They are the third leading cause of death worldwide, accounting for the majority of deaths in the population up to 40 years of age[1] .

Among the types of trauma, spinal cord injury (SCI) is an acute and unexpected event related to growing urbanisation, which has consequences such as an increase in violence and traffic accidents[2,3,4] .

Spinal cord injury (SCI) is defined as an injury to the spine from any external cause, whether or not it affects the spinal cord or nerve roots, in any of its segments[5] . It is a serious disabling syndrome with a variety of signs and symptoms, including pain, changes in sensitivity and motor skills, depending on the vertebral level affected and the degree of involvement of the nervous system[6] .

The injury process in TRM is caused by indirect forces resulting from movements of the trunk and head or by direct aggression on the spinal column[7] . Thus, by direct or indirect action, the primary injury is caused by the transfer of kinetic energy to the spinal cord, causing axons to break and blood vessels to rupture. Local changes resulting from the primary injury, such as haemorrhage, ischaemia of the spinal cord tissue and oedema, can lead to secondary injuries, resulting in an increase in the affected area[8] .

In cases where the spinal cord is compromised, after the trauma there is a period of spinal shock, with loss of all neurological functions in the regions below the level of injury. Hagen et al.[7] state that this period has a variable duration and is characterised by arreflexia, loss of voluntary movement and sensitivity in the body segments innervated below the level of injury.

The return of reflexes indicates the end of the spinal cord shock period, and when this occurs without the return of motor and sensory functions, there is an unfavourable functional prognosis, resulting from a complete or incomplete spinal cord injury[9] .

As well as bodily changes, trauma causes psychosocial changes for the individual[10,11] . The limitations resulting from this trauma, as well as social difficulties, are realities that become present in these people's lives and can interfere with their quality of life[12] .

Treatment for MRI can be done conservatively, through rest, traction and the use of special orthoses, or it can be performed surgically[7] . Surgery is usually indicated in cases of unstable vertebral fractures with spinal cord injury, and prostheses are used to ensure alignment and stabilisation of the spine[13] .

The management of these patients requires a rehabilitation programme involving a multidisciplinary healthcare team[7] . In this process, physiotherapy is considered a key component for an appropriate motor and sensory response ' '[141516] .

The perspectives developed in Neuroscience over the last few decades emphasise the fact that the central nervous system can undergo structural changes as a result of learning[1718] . In this context, the physiotherapist's practice seeks to explore viable skills for the level of impairment of the individual with SCI, following a model of maximising functions by compensating for deficits in motor control, sensitivity and balance[19] . Functional results are targeted according to the level and severity of the injury[15] .

There is a wide variation in the incidence rates of TRM in the world's different geographical regions, but there is clear evidence that developing countries have shown increasing incidence rates in the last decade[20 21] .

In developing countries, the lack of national registry systems and death at the scene of the trauma, as well as in the pre-hospital phase, could explain the lower mortality from SCI in these countries compared to developed countries, where death occurs in the in-hospital phase. Furthermore, in many developing countries there is a diversity or even absence of epidemiological records of SCI.

It is estimated that the incidence of TRM in the United States is between 30 and 40 cases per million inhabitants per year. However, this figure includes an incidence of 8.5% of cases of unknown origin, which may be due to non-traumatic etiologies such as tumours and infections[22] .

In Brazil, retrospective surveys record an incidence of 17.3 cases of MRI per million inhabitants per year, but this figure may be underestimated in a country with more than 200 million inhabitants and a growing concern about road traffic accidents and violence in general[14] .

Data from the Interagency Health Information Network (RIPSA)[23] shows that there has been an increase in traffic accidents since 2000 in the state of Goiás (GO). According to the report, for example, from 2004 to 2012 standardised mortality rates per accident rose from 28 to 31.3 deaths per 100,000 inhabitants, which corresponds to an increase of 12%.

This data can also be seen in a survey carried out by the Programme for the Reduction of Morbidity and Mortality from Traffic Accidents in some of the country's capital cities, in which the city of Goiânia was found to have the highest mortality rates from traffic accidents, especially motorcycling accidents[24] .

According to the records of Seguradora Líder de Danos Pessoais causados por Veículos Automotores de Via Terrestre (DPVAT)[25] , 4.6% of national indemnities to victims of traffic accidents in 2012 were paid in the state of Goiás (GO). Goiás' rate is worrying, given that it accounted for 48.42% of the indemnities in the Centre-West region in the same period.

It's clear that hospital care is essential for delineating the clinical picture of TRM. The type of treatment, the presence of hospital complications and early rehabilitation are determining factors in the patient's prognosis.

Given this situation, this work seeks to answer the question: what are the social and clinical characteristics of patients with TRM treated at a tertiary hospital in Goiás? Based on this theme, we sought to understand the causes and consequences of this condition in the population studied, visualising socioeconomic and health indicators.

Clinically and epidemiologically characterising patients during hospitalisation provides a wealth of information needed to carry out preventive campaigns aimed at the population most vulnerable to this injury.

In addition, information on hospitalisation makes it possible to identify the quality of the service provided, enabling strategies to improve care for these patients, especially with regard to preventing complications, access to rehabilitation and specialised care [',5,21 ',24,26] .

In addition, data on initial hospital costs for this event is essential, as this knowledge allows us to identify actions that need to be optimised in order to reduce costs, eliminate waste and preserve the quality of care provided[27] . In this way, health managers will not only be able to rationalise costs, but also become aware of the importance of this analysis in decision-making, contributing to a better allocation of financial resources in the face of the funding shortfall in the Unified Health System (SUS)[28] .

Studies involving TRM are predominantly descriptive, with a small number of studies establishing interrelationships between variables related to trauma.

Given the above, and the major socio-economic impact of this disease, this book aims to analyse the epidemiology of TRM in patients admitted to the Goiânia Emergency Hospital (HUGO), a reference hospital for high-complexity care in the Midwest region of Brazil.

The objectives of this work are described below:

General objective

To assess the clinical and epidemiological profile of patients with TRM treated at HUGO between 1 January and 31 December 2013.

Specific objectives

- To verify the relationship between the etiology and the sex of the patients;

- To assess the association between the form of treatment for spinal trauma (surgical and conservative), the presence of complications and the length of hospital stay;

- To identify the relationship between the indication for physiotherapy and the presence of motor disability and complications;

- To analyse the association between mortality and the other study variables (gender, age group, vertebral segment affected, presence of spinal cord injury, trauma mechanism and need for admission to the Intensive Care Unit - ICU);

- To evaluate the duration of hospitalisation and the hospital cost of these patients to the SUS.

CHAPTER 2

METHODOLOGY

Type of study

This is a retrospective, descriptive and analytical epidemiological case series study.

Research location

The research was carried out at HUGO, as it is the largest hospital affiliated to the SUS that is able to provide initial care for patients suffering from any type of trauma, and is the main high-complexity reference centre for the whole of the state of Goiás.

HUGO receives patients referred by the Municipal Regulation Centre, the Mobile Emergency Care Service (SAMU), the Fire Brigade and other pre-hospital care services, as well as spontaneous demand.

Inclusion and exclusion criteria

Inclusion criteria were patients admitted to HUGO in 2013, whose medical records contained a descriptive diagnosis of TRM made by an orthopaedic doctor and/or neurosurgeon, confirmed by computed tomography (CT) and/or magnetic resonance imaging (MRI) scans.

Cases whose medical records were not available at the hospital's Medical and Statistical Archive Service (SAME) during data collection were excluded from the study, as were cases of patients who were admitted with a suspicion of the trauma being researched, but whose diagnosis did not correspond to the subject in question.

Data collection

Data was collected from selected medical records using a form designed for this purpose.

The variables identified in the study were: age, gender, marital status, education, occupation, origin, level of injury, aetiology, associated trauma, type of treatment, presence of complications, need for ICU admission, indication for physiotherapy, length of hospitalisation and cost of hospitalisation.

The variables "presence of alcohol intoxication at the time of the injury" and "prescription of physiotherapy after hospital discharge" were excluded because there was no data in the medical records.

To classify the occupation, we used the Brazilian Classification of Occupations (CBO), a simplified version drawn up by the Ministry of Labour and Employment[29] .

The cities of origin of the patients from the interior of the state were grouped by mesoregion, according to the classification drawn up by the Brazilian Institute of Geography and Statistics (IBGE)[30] , which divides the state of GO into 5 mesoregions: Centre, East, North, Northwest and South.

The costs of hospitalisation were obtained from the invoices generated according to the data on the Authorisation for Hospital Admission (AIH) available in each medical record. These invoices express the amount of funds paid by SUS for each hospitalisation.

The complications described during hospitalisation were categorised according to Mello et al.[31] into: complications related to spinal trauma, which would be those described as classic complications of this injury; complications resulting from hospitalisation, which include those acquired in the hospital environment; complications due to associated trauma or previous illnesses, which would be those resulting from the injury, other than the spinal trauma or previous illnesses that the patient had and which were complicated during hospitalisation; as well as surgical complications.

Analysing the data

The data was submitted to descriptive and inferential statistics using the *Statistical Package for the Social Sciences (SPSS)* programme, version 15.0. The chi-square test was used to check for possible associations between the study variables. In 2X2 tables with a small total number of data, the Chi-square test with Fisher's exact significance was used to reduce error.

The median lengths of hospitalisation in the surgical versus conservative treatment groups were compared using the Mann-Whitney test, since the sample distribution in each group was non-normal.

The significance level adopted in this study was 5%.

Ethical aspects

The project was submitted to and approved by the Ethics Committee for Research with Human Beings (CEP) of the State University of Campinas (UNICAMP), under protocol number 182.937.

As this was a study using secondary and retrospective data, the CEP was asked to waive the requirement for a Free and Informed Consent Form (FICF).

There were no conflicts of interest in carrying out this research.

CHAPTER 3

RESULTS

In the case selection phase, around 12,000 medical records were consulted. According to the inclusion criteria defined for this study, 265 cases were identified.

Demographic data

The sociodemographic characterisation of the sample is shown in tables 1 and 2.

The average age of the patients was 32.1 years, ranging from 4 to 87 years, with a median of 36.1 years and a standard deviation of 16.5 years. A ratio of 4.4 men to every woman was found. As for marital status, the "no partner" group, which represented the majority of the sample, included singles, widowers and divorcees. The remaining patients were married or in a stable union, making up the group known as "with a partner". This data, however, was hampered by the lack of information in the medical records (table 1).

Table 1 - Characterisation of TRM by gender, age group and marital status (n=265)

VARIABLE	DISTRIBUTION %(f)
SEX	
Male	81,50% (216)
Female	18,50% (49)
AGE GROUP	
0 to 20 years	18,90% (50)
21 to 30 years old	28,30% (75)
31 to 40 years old	18,10% (48)
41 to 50 years old	12,10% (32)
51 to 60 years old	12,10% (32)
61 years or older	9,40% (25)
Not informed	1,10% (3)
CIVIL STATUS	
No mate	40,75% (108)
With a mate	25,66% (68)
Not informed	38,11% (101)

An even greater loss of information can be seen in the variable called schooling, whose data was present in only 131 of the 265 medical records included in the study (table 2).

Table 2 - Characterisation of TRM by schooling, professional category and origin (n=265)

VARIABLE	DISTRIBUTION % (f)
SCHOOLING	
Primary school	32,83% (87)
High School	13,21% (35)
Higher Education	2,26% (6)
Illiterate	1,13% (3)
Not informed	50,57% (134)

PROFESSIONAL CATEGORY	
Service providers and commerce	37,44% (100)
Students	9,06% (24)
Agricultural workers	7,17% (19)
Administrative Services	4,53% (12)
Pensioners	2,64% (7)
Production and industrial services goods	1,51% (4)
Mid-level technicians	0,75% (2)
Not informed	36,60% (97)
PROCEDURE	
Goiânia metropolitan region	75,10% (199)
Interior of Goiás (GO)	24,10% (64)
Other states in Brazil	0,80% (2)
ORIGIN BY MESOREGION (GO)	N = 263*
Centre	80,99% (213)
South	10,27% (27)
North West	4,94% (13)
North	2,66% (7)
East	0,76% (2)
Not informed	0,38% (1)

'Distribution of GO patients only.

The predominant occupation was service provider and retail worker, followed by student and agricultural worker (table 2). With regard to where the patients came from, the vast majority were from Goiânia and the metropolitan region, although a significant proportion came from the interior of GO. When this data was analysed in terms of distribution by mesoregion, it could be seen that patients from the central region prevailed. With regard to patients from other states, one was from Minas Gerais and the other from the state of Mato Grosso.

Etiology

In terms of aetiology (table 3), traffic accidents predominated, followed by firearm injuries and falls, with the latter two having very close percentages.The only case of spinal injury from diving in shallow waters was a male patient, who died.

Table 3 - Distribution of SCI by trauma aetiology (n=265)

VARIABLE	DISTRIBUTION %(f)
ETIOLOGY	
Traffic accident	40,80% (108)
Firearm injury	22,60% (60)
Falls	22,30% (59)
Hit-and-run	5,30% (14)
Assaults	3,00% (8)
Shallow water diving	0,40% (1)
Other*	4,90% (13)
Not informed	0,80% (2)
FALLS	N = 59**
Roof, bridge, ladder, scaffolding	55,93% (33)
Own height	20,34% (12)

Horse, cart, tree	18,64% (11)
Level***	5,09% (3)
TRAFFIC ACCIDENTS	N = 108****
Motorbike	67,60% (73)
Cars	26,85% (29)
Bicycle	5,55% (6)

'Other: attempted self-extermination, heavy objects falling on the spine or axial trauma.** Distribution of aetiology in relation to types of fall.
***Falls on surfaces below ground level.
""Distribution of traffic accidents according to vehicle.

Falls were categorised according to the reason, with a higher frequency of falls from the roof, bridge, ladder or scaffolding.

Traffic accidents were also divided into subcategories according to the vehicle involved, with a clear predominance of motorbike accidents.

When the association of etiological factors was checked in relation to gender, there was a statistically significant difference in the subcategories of the types of falls (p<0.001) (figure 1), but this difference was not found in relation to the type of traffic accident (p= 0.755) (figure 2).

When we isolate the traumas caused by FAF from the other etiologies and check the association between the prevalence rates by gender, we can see that this was statistically significant, with a prevalence of FAF around two and a half times higher in men than in women (p=0.02) (figure 3).

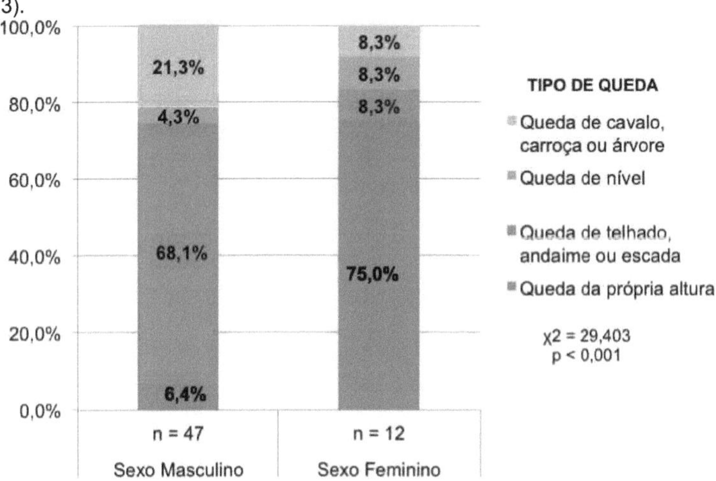

Figura 1 - Distribution of MTR by type of fall, in relation to sex

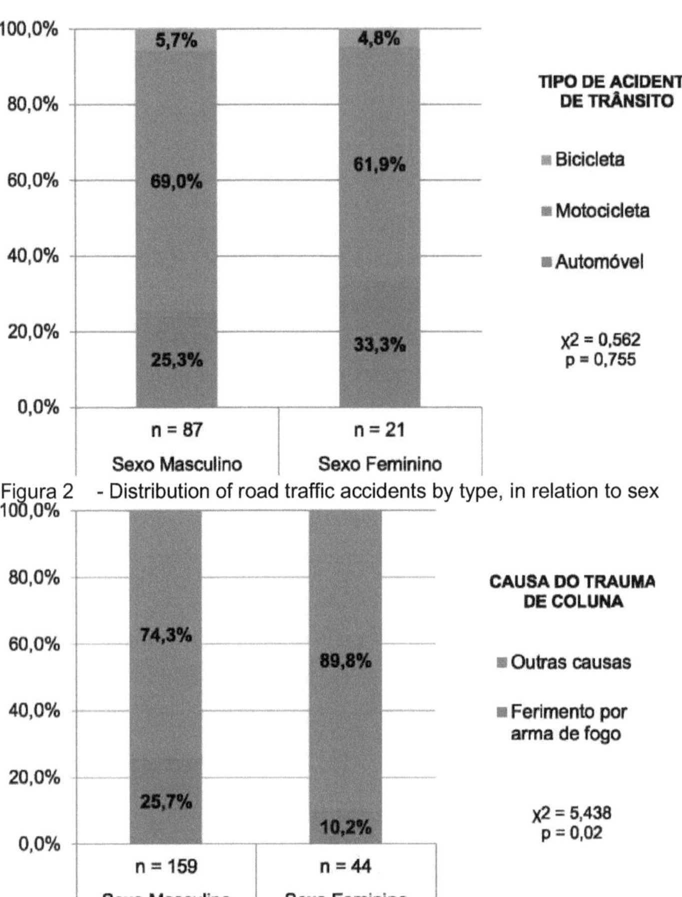

Figura 2 - Distribution of road traffic accidents by type, in relation to sex

Figura 3 - Distribution of firearm-related injuries and other causes, by sex

Clinical data

Table 4 shows the data on the level of vertebrae affected, where it can be seen that trauma to the thoracolumbar spine was predominant.

Table 4 - Distribution of SCI according to vertebral level of trauma and spinal cord involvement (n = 265)

VARIABLE	DISTRIBUTION %(f)
VERTEBRAL LEVEL*	
Upper cervical (C0-C2)	15,85% (42)
Lower cervical (C3-C7)	25,66% (68)
Thoracic (T1-T10)	26,04% (69)
T oracolumbar (T11-L2)	29,43% (78)
Lumbar (L3-L5)	14,34% (38)

SPINAL CORD INJURY	
No injury	50,57% (134)
Complete injury	15,85% (42)
Partial injury	10,94% (29)
No information	22,64% (60)

**Some patients had trauma in more than one region of the spine, so the sum of the percentages is greater than 100%.*

As for neurological impairment, some data was inconclusive due to incomplete information or lack of radiological exams to prove the injury. However, in the medical records, through which this data could be seen, it was observed that the majority of patients did not have a spinal cord injury, and in the cases where this did occur, the complete injury prevailed over the partial injury (table 4).

With regard to motor limitations/disabilities, 52.45% of the patients had some alteration, while 46.42% had no apparent deficits. Three medical records did not show this information (1.13%).

Conservative treatment was the method of choice in 238 cases (89.81%) and surgical intervention was performed in 22 of them (8.30%). The cases in which these data were not in the medical records were those in which the patients received initial treatment and were quickly transferred to another hospital (5 cases =1.89%).

Many patients, however, had associated trauma (174 cases =65.66%), and 109 of these patients underwent surgery for causes not associated with spinal trauma (41.13% of the total sample).

Table 5 shows the distribution of extra-vertebral injuries, with traumatic brain injury (TBI) being the most common.

Table 5 - Distribution of traumas associated with MTR (N=174)

VARIABLE	DISTRIBUTION %(f)
ASSOCIATED TRAUMA*	
Traumatic brain injury	46,55% (81)
Chest trauma	38,50% (67)
Lower limbs	29,88% (52)
Upper limbs	20,69% (36)
Abdominal trauma	19,96% (33)
Other**	22,41% (39)

**Some patients had more than one associated trauma, which is why the percentages add up to more than 100%.*
***Other: trauma to the face, scapula and perineum.*

70 patients (26.42%) needed to be admitted to the ICU, with an average stay of 14 days (minimum of 1 and maximum of 46 days).

Complications

As for complications, 139 patients (52.45%) had them. Patients usually had more than one type of complication, with a total of 395 records (table 6).

Complications related to SCI were the most common, with pain being a complication frequently reported in medical records. Complications due to associated trauma or previous illnesses included pleural effusion and pneumothorax. In terms of complications resulting from hospitalisation, pneumonia was the most common. There were few surgical complications.

When comparing the type of treatment the patient underwent and the presence or absence of complications (figure 4), there was no statistically significant association between the variables, according to the Chi-squared test (p=0.446).

Table 6 - Distribution of types of MTR complications by category (N=139)

VARIABLE	DISTRIBUTION %(f)
Related to spinal trauma*	
Pain	82,01% (114)
Respiratory failure	15,82% (22)
Psychomotor agitation	13,66% (19)
Neurogenic bladder	12,23%(17)
Neurogenic shock	5,75% (8)
Paresthesia	4,32% (6)
Due to associated trauma or previous illnesses	
Pleural effusion	32,37% (45)
Pneumothorax	28,77% (40)
Lowered level of consciousness	20,86% (29)
Epigastralgia	4,32% (6)
Precordialgia	1,44% (2)
As a result of hospitalisation	
Pneumonia	24,46% (34)
Pressure ulcers	7,91% (11)
Septic shock	7,91% (11)
SARA**	7,19% (10)
Urinary tract infection	5,03% (7)
Surgical complications	
Surgical infection	4,32% (6)
Renal insufficiency	4,32% (6)
Tracheoesophageal fistula	1,44% (2)

Some patients had more than one complication, which is why the sum of the percentages is over 100%.
***ARDS: Adult Respiratory Distress Syndrome.*

Physiotherapy

The indication for physiotherapy was reported in 109 medical records (41.13%). Figure 5 shows the distribution of patients who received physiotherapy and the presence or absence of motor disability. Figure 6 shows the cross-referencing of data related to the indication for physiotherapy and the presence of complications. In both cases, a statistical association was found between the variables (p<0.001).

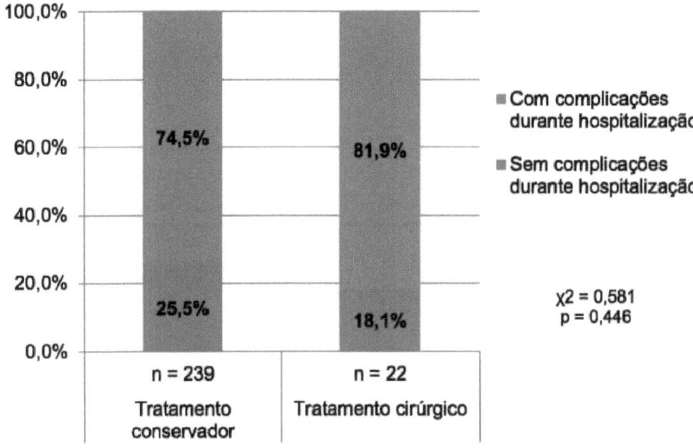

Figura 4 - Distribution of MRT according to type of treatment, by occurrence of complications during hospitalisation

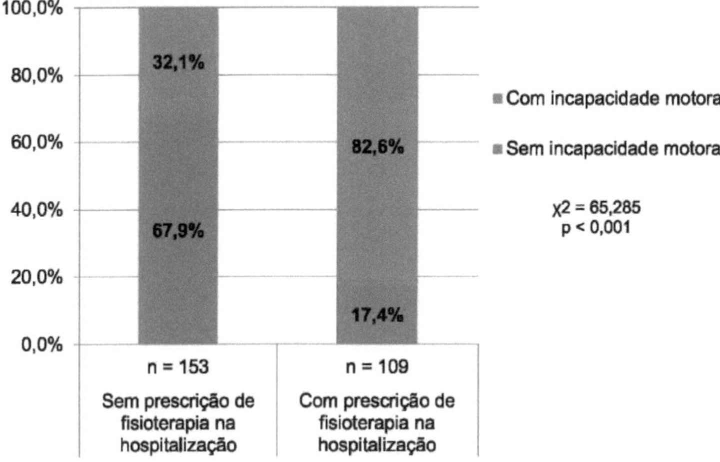

Figura 5 - Distribution ofTRM in terms of indication for physiotherapy, by occurrence of disability/motor limitation

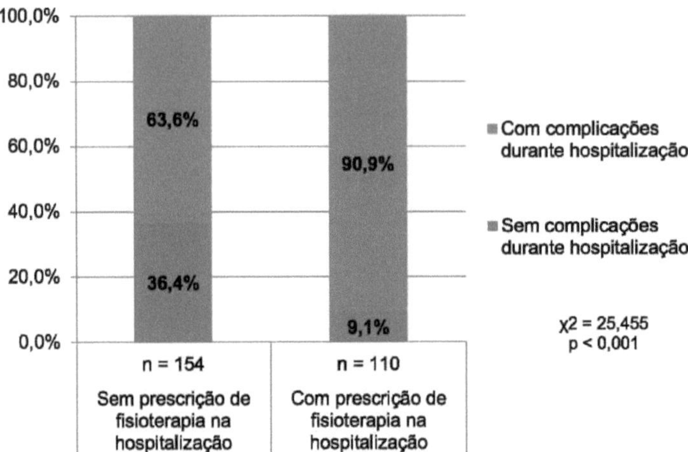

Figura 6 - Distribution of MTR regarding indication for physiotherapy, by occurrence of complications during hospitalisation

Length of hospitalisation

With regard to the length of time patients were hospitalised, the median was 6 days, ranging from 1 to 160 days, and the average was 15 days. When comparing patients who underwent conservative and surgical treatment, the median hospitalisation times were 5 (minimum of 1 and maximum of 160 days) and 15 days (minimum of 4 and maximum of 84), respectively, with a statistically significant difference between the groups (p=0.0001, Mann-Whitney).

Figure 7 shows the data regarding the finalisation of hospital care at the unit surveyed.

Mortality

It can be seen that most patients were discharged and that the case fatality rate was 14%, which is an index that demonstrates disease-specific mortality (figure 7).

The average age of patients who died was 33.5 years, ranging from 4 to 59 years. Other mortality data is shown in Table 7, which shows a statistically significant association between mortality and some sociodemographic and clinical variables.

Alta médica   Transferência   Óbito   Alta administrativa   Evasão

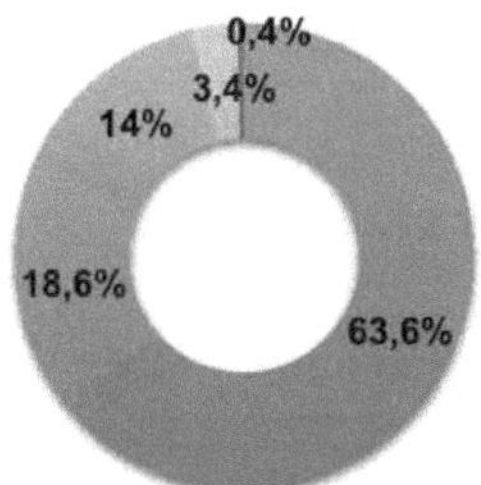

Figura 7 - Distribution of the TRM in terms of the end of hospital care

With regard to the etiology of the trauma, figure 8 shows that although road traffic accidents are quite common (n=89), mortality is higher when the trauma is caused by assaults and being run over (p=0.037).

Cost of hospitalisation

All hospitalisations took place via the SUS. The partial cost of the patients' hospitalisation was R$756,450.37, according to the billing generated from the data on the IHA form. Table 8 shows the details of these amounts, including data by day of hospitalisation.

It's worth noting that the hospital cost of surgical patients does not include plates and screws used to fix the spine, as these materials were not included in the invoices. They are purchased directly by the Goiás State Health Department (SES/GO), with an invoice not available in the medical records.

Table 7 - Distribution of mortality and survival from TRM, by sociodemographic and clinical data (n=265)

VARIABLE	DISTRIBUTION		Chi-squared test *(P)*
	Survivors (N=228) **%(f)**	**Deaths** (N=37) **%(f)**	
SEX			
Male Female	84,70% (182) 91,80% (45)	15,30% (33) 8,20% (04)	*p=0,191*
AGE GROUP			
< 60 years	84,40% (200) 100%	15,60% (37)	*p=0,031**
> 60 years	(25)	0,0% (0)	
SPINAL INJURY			
Cervical	78,20% (79)	21,80% (22)	
Thoracic Lumbar or sacral	91,20% (114) 88,60% (31)	8,80% (11) 11,40% (4)	*p=0,018*
SPINAL CORD INJURY			
No injury Partial injury	92,50% (124)	7,50% (10)	*p=0,0003*

Complete injury	96,60% (28)	3,40% (1)	
	71,40% (30)	28,60% (12)	
ICU HOSPITALISATION			
Yes	53,20 (33)	46,80 (29) 4,00	*p<0,001*
No	96,00 (192)	(8)	

Chi-squared test with Fisher's exact significance.

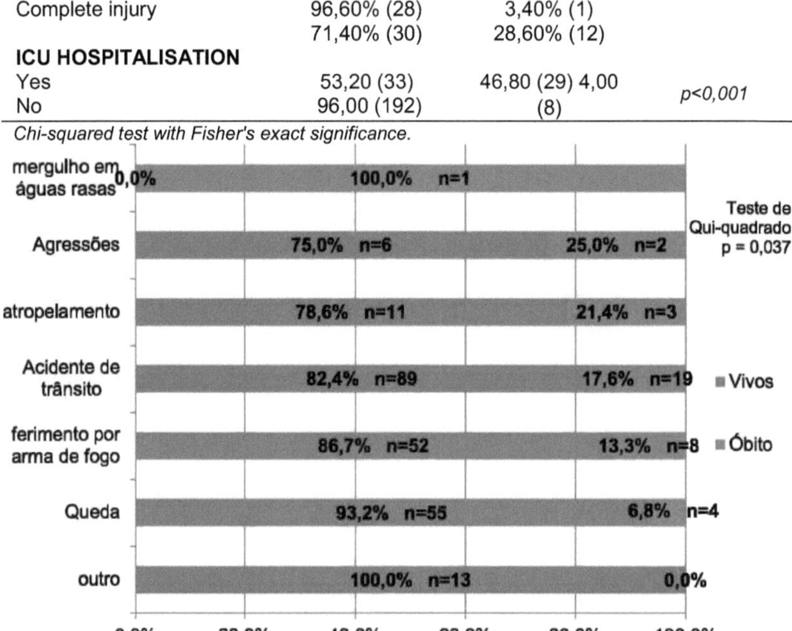

Figura 8 - Distribution of mortality and survival from SCI, by trauma mechanism

Table 8 - Figures for the cost of hospitalisation for 265 patients with SCI

Overall cost of hospitalisation	**VALUE (R$)**
Average	R$ 2.943,57
Standard deviation	R$ 4.868,90
Median	R$ 907,62
Minimum	R$ 192,60
Maximum	R$29.706,10
Cost of hospitalisation per day	**VALUE (R$)**
Average	R$ 257,02
Standard deviation	R$ 342,18
Median	R$ 139,12
Minimum	R$ 14,11
Maximum	R$ 2.794,24

CHAPTER 4

DISCUSSION

Demographic data

The predominance of young male adult victims of SCI is well documented in the literature[4,5,7,26,30,31,32,33]. This was also confirmed in this study, with a male-female ratio of 4.4:1.0 and a mean age of 36.1 years.

Men usually display higher risk behaviour than women, being more exposed to work and recreational activities that predispose them to trauma -[3435]. In addition, they are the main ones involved in violent behaviour[2]. However, Rodrigues et al.[36], Morais[37] and Chamberlain et al.[38] warn about the increase in the incidence of MRI among women in recent times, which reflects cultural and social trends in the changing role of women in society.

The study by Custódio et al.[39], also carried out in a hospital in the city of Goiânia, showed very similar data to the present study, with a higher prevalence in men with a mean age of 35.3 years.

The above represents an important problem, given that this population is in a period of full professional productivity, with their economically active activity interrupted by the injury[4041].

If we look at the low level of education of the subjects in this study, this problem becomes even greater. It is important to emphasise that this finding is repeated in other studies of patients affected by SCI in Brazil, which suggests that this is a national event[3,37,42 43].

Added to this is the fact that the predominant professional occupation in our study was service and trade provider (37.44 per cent), a category with a lower income, usually acquired independently. It is therefore necessary to reflect on the socio-cultural patterns that are perpetuated in the environment studied.

Jácomo and Garcia[43], in a study carried out in the same region of Brazil with victims of SCI due to motorbike accidents, point out that the majority of patients receive social security benefits, but these are not enough to cover all their expenses, and they need to supplement their income with informal activities.

Taking only the age group into consideration, Brito[5], Furlan et al.[20], Jazayeri[22] and Hasler et al.[44] report a bimodal distribution in populations with TRM, with the first prevalence peak in young adults and the second peak being found in elderly individuals. A number of factors can explain the second peak, including osteoporosis due to ageing and a greater predisposition to falls due to the loss of sensory mechanisms and the effects of medication used by this population[45] .

However, in our study this second peak was not observed. This may have been because the average age of the cases in our sample was lower than in the aforementioned studies, and the patients were therefore less subject to the effects of ageing.

As far as origin is concerned, the data shows that HUGO is a benchmark in state hospital care for MTR victims, since many patients came from the interior of Goiás (24.10%). They also suggest the need to create decentralised hospitals, especially in the southern region of the state, where around 10% of the cases came from. In this region there are towns more than 400 kilometres from the capital, which increases the risk of morbidity and mortality in transport to HUGO.

With regard to marital status, there was a predominance of patients without a partner (40.75%), which can also be seen in the study by Blanes et al.[46] , carried out in the city of São Paulo, which identified more than half of the sample made up of single individuals (61.70%). The study by Santiago et al.[47] , carried out in the north-eastern region of Brazil, also showed this predominance (37.50%).

Etiology

With regard to aetiology, the findings are similar to those found by Sothmann et al.[26] , DeVivo[48] , Rahimi-Movaghar et al.[49] and Barras and Basso[50] , in which road traffic accidents appear to be the main cause of TRM.

Lee et al.[21] , in a study that sought to map the epidemiology of road traffic accidents around the world, stated that the number of traffic accidents is decreasing or remaining stable in developed countries. However, the authors showed that this rate is growing alarmingly in developing countries, due to the increase in the number and power of vehicles, the precariousness of the road network infrastructure in these places, as well as the challenge of enforcing traffic laws.

Goiânia has been labelled one of the Brazilian capitals with the most violent traffic in the country[37] . The probable causes for this are numerous. In addition to the issues mentioned by Lee et al.[21] , the capital of GO is a city with wide, flat streets, which makes it easier for vehicles to accelerate.

According to the report by the National Institute of Science and Technology[51] , between 2001 and 2012, the composition of the motor vehicle fleet in Goiânia changed substantially, especially in favour of motorbikes. The same report states that the Centre-West region had a motorisation rate of 29.4 cars/100 inhabitants, above the national average of 25.9 cars/100 inhabitants. This information may explain the high frequency of TRM due to traffic accidents in this sample (40.80 per cent), affecting both men and women, with no statistically significant relationship with gender.

The number of accidents involving motorbikes (67.60 per cent) is noteworthy. It is a fact that motorcyclists are more at risk of dying or suffering bodily injury than car occupants[3 52] . Oliveira et al.[53] found, for example, that patients with SCI due to motorbike accidents are generally male, young and have high rates of neurological deficit.

One factor that may be related to this mode of transport and trauma is the dynamic functioning and structure of the motorbike, which does not have an adequate protection system[2454] . Added to this is the risky behaviour of drivers, which increases the likelihood of accidents[55] .

You also have to consider that motorbikes are less expensive than cars, both in terms of purchase and maintenance '[535456] . Furthermore, in the Goiânia region there is a predominance of dry weather and few inclines in the streets, which further contributes to the increase in the fleet.

In contrast to our data, Leal Filho et al.[4] , Brito et al.[5] , Anderle et al.[33] and Rodrigues et al.[36] described falls as the main etiological factor in SCI. In these cases, however, the age range of the sample studied was higher than in our sample. Furthermore, these studies were carried out in the south-eastern and north-eastern regions of Brazil, where the practice of irregular constructions used for celebratory gatherings (slabs) is quite common.

Even in international studies, such as those by Wu et al.[40] and Guzelkuçuk et al.[45] , there has been an increase in the prevalence of falls in the elderly. However, it should be borne in mind that this occurs mainly in developed countries, where there is a continuous increase in population ageing.

When the type of fall was stratified, it can be seen that women are more likely to suffer falls from their own height, while men have a higher risk of falling from the roof, scaffolding or ladders, a fact that can be explained by the occupational hazard related to activities such as construction.

Another etiological finding in this study that deserves to be discussed is the high frequency of trauma due to FAF (22.60%). The results showed a statistically significant difference between the sexes when compared to other causes, with a clear higher prevalence in males. This result corroborates research by Araújo Júnior et al.[2] , Sothmann et al.[26] , Blanes et al.[46] , Santiago et al.[47] , Tugcu et al.[57] , Carvalho and Saraiva[58] , in which South African and Latin American countries, especially Brazil, are highlighted for their high rates of violence among civil society, causing great social concern.

Pimentel et al.[59] concluded that TRM caused by FAF causes serious, irreversible sequelae, with incalculable damage to the quality of life of its victims and high costs for the government.

In this context, Barras and Basso[50] state that the growing urbanisation of the Midwest region of the country, where Goiânia is located, highlights the fact that the clinical and epidemiological characteristics of TRM are influenced by local culture, industrialisation and violence.

As Touno said[60] , the problem of violence, in its most varied forms, involves aspects that go beyond the remit of the health sector. However, it's not hard to see that it's this sector that bears the brunt of the problem, since it's the one that receives and treats victims of TRM.

As for the other aetiological findings in this study, table 3 shows that being run over and assaults accounted for 8.30% of the causes. Diving in shallow waters occurred in only one patient (0.40%) and the other causes included, among other things, attempts at self-extermination (4.90%).

Clinical data

Vertebral level affected

In terms of injured vertebral segments, thoracolumbar trauma was predominant (T11-L2=29.43%), followed by thoracic (T1-T10=26.04%) and lower cervical (C3-C7=25.66%). However, if we consider the sum of the frequencies of injuries in the upper cervical (15.85%) and lower cervical (25.66%) regions, the cervical region as a whole is the most prevalent (41.51%).

Stein et al.[9] state that spinal injuries tend to occur in areas of greater mobility. In this regard, Karimi[61] adds that the thoracolumbar region is more susceptible to injury due to the abrupt change from the fixed segment of the spine (costal gradient) to the mobile segment (lumbar spine).

In the study by Custódio et al.[39] , with etiological factors very similar to those in this study, the site of greatest involvement in the spine was the thoracic region (54.80%). Barros and Basso[50] also identified a higher prevalence of thoracolumbar injuries in TRM, with 51% of individuals with injuries in this region. However, depending on the study, this topography may vary.

The results of Fernandes et al.[62] showed that the most affected vertebrae were L1 to L5 (15.80%), C1 to C7 (12.50%) and T1 to T12 (9.80%).

Morais et al.[42] and Bernardi[63] describe a predominance of cervical injuries in SCI. These authors suggest that road traffic accidents lead to a higher rate of injury in this region, while falls have a higher frequency of thoracolumbar injuries. In our study, this was confirmed, since road traffic accidents were the main cause and falls were also quite frequent.

It is important to remember that several patients in this study had more than one spinal injury, which may be related to the severity of the traumas, especially traffic accidents, which are high-energy traumas.

Spinal cord involvement

With regard to spinal cord involvement, despite the high frequency of inconclusive data (22.64%), the results showed a predominance of cases without this involvement (50.57%). However, in the cases with involvement, the complete lesion (15.85%) outweighed the incomplete lesion (10.94%). This clinical finding was also reported in the systematic review carried out by Rahimi-Movaghar et al.[49] , which included 64 scientific studies from 28 countries around the world.

It is known that when TRM affects nerve structures, patients suffer impairment of their motor, sensory and autonomic functions, with major repercussions on their activities of daily living[37] .

Treatment for TRM

The treatment adopted for TRM was predominantly conservative (89.81%), using classic methods such as bed rest, traction and stabilisation with orthoses (waistcoats).

The choice of conservative treatment was based on the absence of neurological damage or unstable fractures, or on unfavourable clinical conditions for the invasive procedure.

Surgical treatment was carried out in 8.30 per cent of patients and consisted of implanting screws and an internal fixator, as well as removing the projectile in some cases of FAF. Root decompression for pain relief was also necessary in some cases.

According to Tavares et al.[34] , Rodrigues et al.[36] , Rahimi-Movaghar[49] and Wyndaele and Wyndaele[64] , around 15 to 20% of cases of TRM require surgical treatment.

Lenehan et al.[65] , in a Canadian population study, showed that there was a greater tendency towards surgical treatment during the 10-year follow-up period (1995 to 2004). However, the authors did not observe concomitant changes in mortality rates or even a reduction in the length of time patients were hospitalised.

Associated traumas

The presence of associated trauma is frequent in cases of SCI, especially when the most common etiologies are traffic accidents, falls and FAF. This is because they are high-impact events, which usually culminate in multiple injuries[42 66] .

This finding was confirmed in the present study. 174 patients had associated trauma (65.66%), and surgical intervention was required to treat these injuries in 109 cases (41.13%).

When looking at the most frequent extra-vertebral traumas (TBI, chest trauma and lower limb trauma), the relationship between the associated injuries and the main aetiologies found in this study is clear.

According to Macciocchi et al.[67] , the incidence of TBI associated with SCI varies depending on the diagnostic markers used in each study. For studies using the International Classification of Diseases (ICD), these authors report an incidence of 16% to 24% of concomitant occurrence of these two diseases. In our sample, the frequency of TBI was much higher than this figure (46.55%), which may indicate the greater severity of the accidents, which would have led to more serious injuries. Yang et al.[66] , in a study carried out in China, found a relationship between the presence of associated injuries and the severity of the cases.

As previously mentioned, the other associated traumas are related to the high rate of road traffic accidents, especially those involving motorcyclists, which usually result in injuries to the chest and lower limbs.

Motor limitation/incapacity

Motor impairment was reported in approximately half of the medical records (50.96%). However, it was difficult to classify the degree of disability based on the medical records available, as there was not always a neurological examination to quantify the impairment.

Assessment scales scientifically labelled as the gold standard in the assessment of TRM[14] , such as the *American Spinal Injury Association (ASIA) scale,* Frankel and the Functional Independence Measure (FIM), were not routinely used in the service, reducing the objectivity of the test.

In this way, the patients who had some disability could have anything from a functional limitation due to pain, without necessarily having a neurological impairment, to a spinal cord injury.

Rieder[14] and Touno[60] state that in cases of cervical injury, the incidence of functional impairment is much higher, as the spinal cord is more exposed and susceptible to rupture in this segment, as well as the mechanisms of cervical trauma being more aggressive.

On the other hand, Kumar et al.[68] showed, through a study that followed patients with cervical SCI for 6 weeks, that 20.00% of patients with complete spinal cord injury showed signs of functional recovery and 56.36% of these showed no signs of recovery during this period. Of the patients with incomplete injuries, 69.01% showed signs of recovery, while 25.35% showed no signs at all.

This analysis brings us back to the fact that, in addition to physical repercussions, MTR has economic and social consequences for the community, since many patients with this condition are also affected by the disease.

This type of trauma requires specialised help, some of them for the rest of their lives.

Intensive Care Unit

ICU support was necessary in 26.42 per cent of patients. The causes were varied and the indication occurred mainly in patients with polytrauma.

The average length of stay for patients in the ICU was 14 days, which leads us to consider that complex cases were referred to this unit.

Bertoncello et al.[52] , Sousa et al[69] and Kucukdurmaz and Alijanipour[70] justify that multiple traumas require several treatments, which increases the risk of complications and consequently makes the patient more unstable, leading them to need intensive care.

According to Santos et al.[71] , the greater the severity of the neurological involvement, the greater the chance of the patient suffering complications and requiring ICU admission. These researchers also state that neurological status after trauma is the most important risk factor in determining morbidity and mortality in these patients.

Complications

Complications during hospitalisation were recorded in 139 patients (52.45%), but some of them had more than one type of complication, totalling 395 records.

Grossman et al.[72] reported this problem in approximately 57% of patients, corroborating the data from our study. Santos et al.[71] , on the other hand, identified fewer complications and found them in 45% of the sample studied.

The most common complications observed in our study were MRI-related, with pain being the most frequent (82.01%). Among the complications resulting from hospitalisation, pneumonia (24.46%), pressure ulcers and septic shock (7.91% each) predominated. This result differs from the literature in general, which identifies a higher proportion of cases of hospitalisation-related complications, such as urinary tract infection and pressure ulcers, as observed in the studies by Mello et al.[31] , Morais[37] and Rahimi-Movaghar et al.[49] . This difference in our results can be attributed to the fact that HUGO is a hospital that provides initial care to trauma victims, and the patient is therefore in the acute phase of the event, when these complications have not yet set in.

Lindgren et al.[73] state that, in general, approximately 40% of patients with TRM develop pressure ulcers while still hospitalised. This suggests that some complications may have gone unrecorded in our study because they were not clearly stated in the medical records. For example, in some medical records there was a record of "fever", but no infectious focus described; in other cases, there was a medical prescription for a dressing, but no mention of the presence of a pressure ulcer.

Chopra et al.[74] showed a statistically significant difference in hospital costs and mortality between patients with infected and non-infected pressure ulcers, demonstrating the importance of assessing this complication.

It is worth noting that pressure ulcers are complications with a higher incidence in patients undergoing surgical procedures, as immobility and the appearance of moisture due to the use of drains, wound secretion and perspiration are risk factors for the development of this complication[75] .

In our sample, surgical procedures were infrequent, which may have contributed to reducing the development of this complication in the short term. It should also be noted that this type of complication (resulting from hospitalisation) is preventable.

Urinary tract infections, for example, can be prevented by measures such as intermittent catheterisation or bladder emptying manoeuvres[76] . Pressure ulcers can be prevented by keeping the skin intact, dry and moisturised, using egg crate mattresses, changing position every two hours, protecting the skin at pressure points and removing the patient from the bed[75] .

With regard to respiratory complications, these can be prevented with respiratory physiotherapy, proper positioning and guidance given to the patient and carers during feeding, avoiding choking which predisposes to aspiration pneumonia -[3763] .

Therefore, the effectiveness of protective and preventive measures can be considered an indicator of the quality of the service -[7277] .

With regard to complications due to associated trauma, pleural effusion (32.37%), pneumothorax (28.77%) and lowered level of consciousness (20.86%) stood out. These complications are clearly related to the associated trauma, once again reflecting the severity of the events.

Surgical complications were less frequent in our study. Surgical wound infection and secondary renal failure were reported with the same frequency (4.32% of cases). Tracheoesophageal fistula was seen in only 2 patients (1.44%).

In the clinical-epidemiological study carried out at the Bahia General Hospital by Fernandes et al.[62] , surgical wound infection was observed in only 1.20% of complications. The authors relate the low occurrence of this complication to the appropriate standard precaution measures and hand hygiene by healthcare professionals and companions, as well as the effectiveness of sterilisation and handling of surgical materials and the surgical environment.

It is interesting to add that Grossman et al.[72] showed in their study that half of the total number of complications in patients with SCI occurs in the first week of hospitalisation. In turn, Morais et al.[78] point out that patients with complications remain in hospital for longer and have a higher risk of dying.

When comparing the type of treatment the patient underwent and the presence of complications (figure 4), there was no statistically significant difference between the groups of patients treated conservatively and surgically (p=0.446).

Yang et al.[66] state that there is a relationship between treatment options and injury severity, with surgery being a common intervention for patients with high functional risk injuries. In addition, this procedure prevents new spinal cord injuries from occurring.

The treatment of TRM has changed in recent years. Advances in instrumentation, anaesthesia and biomaterials, as well as the increased life expectancy of individuals, have increased the choice of surgical treatment[79] .

The study by Thompson et al.[13] , published in 2016, concludes that early surgery in individuals with SCI, when carefully indicated, can optimise neurological recovery and reduce patient complications, reducing the time and costs of hospitalisation. Bourassa-Moreau et al.[80] even suggested that patients with SCI should be operated on before 24 hours after the injury to ensure lower morbidity and mortality.

Physiotherapy

It is true that some patients with SCI require immobilisation of the spine. However, this condition does not imply absolute rest or contraindicate physiotherapy[16] . This study, however, found that this indication only occurred in around 41 per cent of patients.

Musienko et al.[81] and Boland et al.[82] have provided us with scientific evidence that proves the efficiency of functional treatment in the rehabilitation process of patients with TRM. According to Harvey[15] and Galea et al.[83] , techniques based on motor learning and control are the most effective.

In addition, performing global exercises is also important, as it prevents systemic deleterious effects, including the correction of postural derangements that compromise the ventilatory mechanics of these patients ['8485 86] . These consequences are devastating, which further emphasises the need for early rehabilitation[60 ' '6872 ' '8788] .

Respiratory physiotherapy is based on the use of scientifically proven techniques aimed at maintaining and/or re-establishing the patient's ventilatory mechanics. This involves using resources aimed at lung re-expansion, improving alveolar ventilation and increasing functional residual capacity[16 89] . In some cases, bronchial hygiene manoeuvres and assisted coughing techniques are used to maintain airway patency[90] . In addition, respiratory physiotherapy strengthens the remaining ventilatory muscles and improves cardiorespiratory conditioning, which promotes cardiovascular protection and increases patient survival[91,92,93] .

Early physiotherapy care has been linked to a good functional prognosis for the patient. Scivoletto et al.[94] advocate starting rehabilitation as soon as possible, as soon as there are no medical or orthopaedic contraindications to doing so. These authors carried out a study with 150 patients with TRM divided into three groups according to whether they started rehabilitation early, mid-term or late, and found a significant difference in functionality in patients who underwent early rehabilitation.

Wuermser et al.[95] also suggest that this type of intervention should start as early as possible because delays can adversely affect the patient's functional recovery.

In turn, Andresen et al.[96] state that physiotherapy leads to greater control of the patient's morbidities, such as pain and spasticity, bringing benefits that have a positive impact on their quality of life.

The assessment of the association between the indication for physiotherapy and the presence of motor limitations/disabilities proved to be statistically significant ($p<0.001$) and it is therefore important to note that 49 patients (32.10%) had motor limitations/disabilities and yet did not receive this specialised care (figure 5). Another fact to consider is that the patients who did receive specialised care were predominantly those who already had complications ($p<0.001$) (figure 6).

This modest role for hospital physiotherapy is not exclusive to the hospital studied. Campos et al.[97] , in a study aimed at investigating the criteria used by neurologists to refer patients for physiotherapy, found that although most doctors refer their patients, only half of them believe in the effectiveness of the treatment. The authors showed that the referral of physiotherapy was related to the doctor's greater clinical experience, i.e. their greater contact with the positive results of the intervention, rather than their scientific knowledge of its effectiveness. Thus, the authors concluded that there is a need for physiotherapists to disseminate scientific evidence to support the referral of patients.

Jorge et al.[98] also noted that medical requests for follow-up by the hospital physiotherapy team occurred in only 1% of cases, and that these referrals were predominantly for respiratory physiotherapy. The authors pointed out that rehabilitation in the majority of general hospitals seems to be less than ideal and shows a lack of training for rehabilitation teams in the wards. Changing this reality requires institutional effort and continuous work to promote the multidisciplinary team.

It is worth noting, however, that in places where there are rehabilitation centres, as is the case in Goiânia, patients are transferred directly from emergency hospitals to these centres as soon as they become clinically stable. This allows for earlier intervention by the multidisciplinary team, which is extremely important for preventing secondary complications and improving the patient's quality of life[12] ". However, a proportion of these patients do not receive specialised treatment due to a lack of places in these centres. In our sample, we found that 49 patients (18.60 per cent) were transferred from HUGO to the city's rehabilitation hospital, leaving a proportion of them without access to this service.

Length of hospitalisation

In our sample, the average length of hospitalisation was 15 days. Similar data was found by Creôncio et al.[100] , in which this period comprised 17.8 days. In the study by Pereira and Jesus[101] , the average was slightly higher, at 23 days.

According to Hagen[102] , this time varies between hospital units and is much longer in specialised rehabilitation centres, with an average of 67 days.

Touno[60] describes that the average length of hospital stay has increased over the years, with the level of injury and degree of spinal cord involvement affecting the length of stay, with an average of 10 days for cervical injuries, while for thoracic or sacral injuries the average hospital stay is 8 days.

When comparing patients undergoing surgical and conservative treatment, the findings of this study show that hospitalisation time is longer when surgical intervention is necessary (around 10 days longer). This suggests that the length of hospitalisation also depends on the type of treatment selected. Some factors may be responsible for this, such as the delay in carrying out tests, the unavailability of the operating theatre or even materials such as plates and screws to fix the fracture immediately. This was observed in the medical records through medical progressions: "awaiting surgery" or "awaiting CT scan to programme surgery", "awaiting material for procedure", among others.

Another observation that deserves to be highlighted is the fact that hospitalisation of patients with SCI is often relatively quick at the time of the trauma event, but due to the secondary impairments that patients may present, there is a greater risk that they will require further hospitalisations throughout their lives, with longer lengths of stay in these cases[103104] .

As for the outcome of the study, the majority of patients were discharged from hospital (63.60 per cent), and in these cases the nursing team provided guidance to the patient and the family on how to care for the patient. Cases that were being monitored by a physiotherapist also received specific guidance from this professional.

In addition to this outcome, 3.40 per cent of patients were administratively discharged, which is the hospital's prerogative in cases where discharge was requested by the patient themselves or by family members or friends. In this case, the procedure was authorised by a specialist doctor, who had previously assessed the risks and collected the signature of the patient or their legal guardian on the specific consent form for this purpose.

There were also evasions (0.40%), which were cases in which the patient left the hospital without medical authorisation and without informing the department where the patient was staying.

49 patients (18.60 per cent) were transferred to other hospital units because they had private medical insurance or even to follow up at the rehabilitation hospital, as mentioned in the previous section.

Mortality

Mortality in our series was 14%, which coincides with the upper limit of what is found in the literature for acute TRM events, which ranges from 4.9% to 14 2%[7 '20,21] .[22 '49 ' ' '72781] oo. 102

The relationship between mortality and the variables in this study showed that death is higher when the trauma occurs in individuals under the age of 60. This result corroborates the data found by Lalwani et al.[105] , who describe the group aged between 25 and 64 as being the most susceptible to death from SCI.

Cervical spine involvement, the presence of spinal cord injury and the need for ICU support were also identified as factors associated with higher mortality from SCI (Table 7).

Morais et al.[42] , Neumann et al.[106] , as well as Saunders et al.[107] , also describe the severity of the injury as a significant factor, with cervical involvement and complete spinal cord injury having a greater chance of in-hospital mortality, as they are more disabling injuries and susceptible to greater complications.

Another significant finding is that 33 patients who died were male, while only 4 were female. Although there was no statistically significant difference, the data suggests that, as well as being less frequent, trauma in women causes less aggressive injuries.

As for aetiology, figure 8 shows a relationship between the mechanism of trauma and mortality, with p=0.037. Although the main aetiology of SCI is related to road traffic accidents, FAF and falls, there is a higher mortality rate due to aggression and pedestrian accidents, with worrying rates.

Souza[35] leads us to conclude that violence is a determining factor in youth mortality. In Brazil, these issues are exacerbated by intense inequalities and other adverse conditions for citizenship.

Cost of hospitalisation

The cost of hospital treatment demonstrates the initial economic impact of TRM.

It is a fact that patients arriving at hospital units with this type of trauma present a significant degree of complexity, with a risk of death and the need for complex care[62 71] .

In view of this, it is possible to consider that length of stay is linked to survival time and the complexity of the patient's illnesses. This set of factors then defines the cost of hospitalisation[108] .

Due to the large variations in costs found in this study, with a high standard deviation, the median is the data that best represents the sample (R$907.62). However, when comparing the average (R$2,943.57) with studies by other authors, the costs found in this study are higher. Santos et al.[109] , for example, report an average cost of R$ 653.79 per hospitalisation for MRT in state hospitals in Rio de Janeiro.

Touno[60] describes that the average cost of hospitalisations resulting from spinal fractures in Brazil in 2005 was R$1,318.85, although this figure varies significantly when there is a spinal cord injury and in cases of injuries to the cervical vertebrae. The higher number of patients with neurological impairment and longer length of stay in our sample may explain this higher average cost.

It is worth pointing out that in Brazil, public resources for the health sector are scarce. The spending profile for care in this sector is at a level that does not match the reality of costs, and is far from what happens in the Brazilian private sector, and even further from the amounts spent for this purpose in developed countries[27] . Furthermore, the reimbursement amounts practised by the SUS only cover part of the costs of hospital services.

Marinho et al.[28] discussed the underfunding of the SUS and showed a significant difference between the real value and the amount paid by the SUS for highly complex procedures. These aspects reinforce the need to create cost centres so that the revision of the SUS table can be closer to reality, as the underfunding of treatments has prognostic implications for patients.

In addition, it is necessary to consider that when SCI results in spinal cord injury, there is a need for multi-professional follow-up throughout life, and the costs identified in this study are only the initial ones with this injury[100] .

Limitations of the study

This study had some limitations and difficulties, such as: (1) it was difficult to locate cases of TRM, as the medical records were searched manually; (2) medical records had incomplete or scarce data, (3) there was a lack of standardisation in the clinical records of these individuals and (4) the medical records were stored inadequately in a damp, poorly ventilated place, making them sensitive to handling.

It should be noted that we used secondary data, collected retrospectively, which prevents us from carrying out more in-depth multivariate analyses.

In addition, the quality of the information can vary according to the level of management, in terms of the accuracy of the information in the medical records and the completion of the AIH.

It should also be emphasised that neuroimaging is an indispensable tool for determining the initial diagnosis of patients with SCI. However, HUGO did not have enough technical and human resources to deal with all the demand directed to it. As such, the number of cases in this study may have been underestimated.

However, considering the ecological effect of the information, we believe that the analysis carried out is appropriate for the type of inference that this research set out to make.

CHAPTER 5

CONCLUSION

In view of the results found, TRM proved to be an important cause of morbidity and mortality in the population studied.

There was a higher frequency of trauma in young, male individuals, without partners, with low levels of schooling, working in services and commerce, from the capital of the state of Goiás or its metropolitan region.

Traffic accidents proved to be the main cause of trauma, particularly motorbike accidents. Another important cause was FAF, which was more common in men. Falls were also an important cause, with men falling more often from roofs, scaffolding or ladders, while women fell more often from their own height.

The most affected vertebral level was the thoracolumbar, but when the levels were considered separately, the cervical lesion was numerically higher. Most of the patients had no spinal cord involvement.

The treatment of choice for the vast majority of cases was conservative and did not require hospitalisation in the LTCU. More than half of the patients had an associated injury, with TBI being the most common type. More than half of the sample also had some motor limitation.

The most commonly reported complications were pain, pleural effusion, pneumothorax and pneumonia, and there was no significant relationship between the presence of complications and the type of treatment the patient underwent.

Physiotherapy was used for just under half of the patients, and the indication was mainly for patients with motor disabilities and complications that had already set in, which explains the need for an increase in this team at the hospital studied, as well as greater multidisciplinary integration for patient rehabilitation.

Hospitalisation lasted an average of 15 days, and was longer for surgical patients. The partial costs of treating the 265 patients with MRT were low, suggesting that they were not in line with the reality of costs, and that the SUS was therefore underfunding the public hospital.

Mortality was 14 per cent and the factors associated with the highest prevalence of death were age under 60, the presence of trauma to the cervical spine, complete spinal cord injury and the etiology of the trauma.

The descriptive and analytical nature of this research not only made it possible to characterise the variables associated with TRM in the region studied, but also contributed to the planning of actions by health managers in the state of Goiás.

It should be emphasised, however, that more detailed information on the main etiologies should be continually carried out so that preventive intervention can be generated according to the needs of the region. Firearms control measures must also be carried out more effectively, as well as an understanding of the nature of the social problems that generate violence, which could reduce these TRM rates in our society.

In conclusion, it is necessary to consider the need for a national registry to notify cases of SCI. This registry is fundamental for understanding the epidemiology and, consequently, for preventing this health problem, since the only way to improve the population's quality of life and reduce costs for these patients is to prevent traumas and complications from occurring.

CHAPTER 6

REFERENCES

1. Parreira JG, Matar MR, Torres ALB, Perlingeiro JAG, Solda SC, Assef JC. Comparative analysis of injuries identified in victims of falls from a height and other closed trauma mechanisms. Rev Col Bras Cir. 2014;41(4):272-7.
2. De Araújo Júnior FA, Heinrich CB, Cunha MLV, Veríssimo DCA, Rehder R, Pinto CAS, et al. Spinal cord trauma due to firearm projectile injury: epidemiological evaluation. Coluna/Columna. 2011;10(4):290-2.
3. Diniz IV, Soares RAS, Do Nascimento JA, Soares MJGO. Characterisation of Traffic Accident Victims with Spinal Cord Injury. R Bras Ci Saúde. 2012;16(3):371-8.
4. Leal Filho MB, Borges G, De Almeida BR, Aguiar ADAX, Vieira MADCES, Dantas KDS, et al. Spinal cord injury: Epidemiologycal study of 386 cases with emphasis on those patients admitted more than four hours after the trauma. Arq Neuropsiquiatr. 2008;66(2B):365-8.
5. Brito LMO, Chein MBC, Marinho SC, Duarte TB. Epidemiological assessment of patients with spinal cord injury. Rev Col Bras Cir. 2011 ;38(5):304-9.
6. Cunha MLV, Cunha LV, Veríssimo DCA, Rehder R, Borba LAB. Epidemiological study of spinal fractures in a reference centre for spinal pathology in Paraná. Arq Bras Neurocir. 2012;31 (4): 179-83.
7. Hagen EM, Rekand T, Gilhus NE, Gronning M. Traumatic spinal cord injuries incidence, mechanisms and course. Tidsskr Nor Laegeforen. 2012; 132(7):831-7.
8. Lee-Kubli CA, Ingves M, Henry KW, Shiao R, Collyer E, Tuszynski MH, et al. Analysis of the behavioural, cellular and molecular characteristics of pain in severe rodent spinal cord injury. Exp NeuroL 2016;278:91-104.
9. Stein DM, Pineda JA; Roddy V, Knight WA. Emergency neurological life support: traumatic spine injury. Neurocrit Care. 2015;23(2):155-64.

10. Craig A, Perry KN, Guest R, Tran Y, Dezarnaulds A, Hales A, et al. Prospective Study of the occurrence of psychological disorders and comorbidities after spinal cord injury. Arch Phys Med Rehabil. 2015;96(8): 1426- 34.
11. Lude P, Kennedy P, Elfstrom ML, Ballert CS. Quality of Life in and After Spinal Cord Injury Rehabilitation: a longitudinal multicentre study. Top Spinal Cord Inj Rehabil. 2014;20(3): 197-207.
12. Brunozi AE, Silva AC, Gonçalves LF, Veronezi RJB. Quality of life in traumatic spinal cord

injury. Rev Neurocienc. 2011 ;19(1):139-44.

13. Thompson C, Feldman DE, Mac-Thiong JM. Surgical management of patients following traumatic spinal cord injury: identifying barriers to early surgery in a specialised spinal cord injury centre. J Spinal Cord Med. 2016;39(3): in press.

14. Rieder MDM. Spinal cord trauma: epidemiological, functional recovery and molecular biology aspects [PhD Thesis]. Porto Alegre (RS): Federal University of Rio Grande do Sul; 2014.

15. Harvey LA. Physiotherapy rehabilitation for people with spinal cord injuries. J Physiother. 2016;62(1):4-11.

16. Chu J, Harvey LA, Ben M, Batty J, Avis A, Adams R. Physical therapists' ability to predict future mobility after spinal cord injury. J Neurol Phys Ther. 2012;36(1):3-7.

17. Jacobi A, Bareyre FM. Regulation of axonal remodelling following spinal cord injury. Neural Regen Res. 2015; 10(10): 1555-7.

18. Hansen CN, Faw TD, White S, Buford JA, Grau JW, Basso DM. Sparing of descending axons rescues interneuron plasticity in the lumbar cord to allow adaptive learning after thoracic spinal cord injury. Front. Neural Circuits. 2016: in press.

19. Roy RR, Harkema SJ, Edgerton VR. Basic concepts of activity-based interventions for improved recovery of motor function after spinal cord injury. Arch Phys Med Rehabil. 2012;93(9): 1487-97.

20. Furlan JC, Sakakibara BM, Miller WC, Krassioukov AV. Global incidence and prevalence of traumatic spinal cord injury. Can J Neurol Sei. 2013;40(4):456-64.

21. Lee BB, Cripps RA, Fitzharris M, Wing PC. The global map for traumatic spinal cord injury epidemiology: update 2011, global incidence rate. Spinal Cord. 2014;52(2): 110-6.

22. Jazayeri SB, Beygi S, Shokraneh F, Hagen EM, Rahimi-Movaghar V. Incidence of traumatic spinal cord injury worldwide: a systematic review. Eur Spine J. 2015;24(5):905-18.

23. Brazil. Interagency Health Information Network (RIPSA). Indicators and basic data (IDB). Brasília; 2012.

24. Souza ER, Minayo MCS, Franco LG. Evaluation of the process of implantation and implementation of the Traffic Accident Morbidity and Mortality Reduction Programme. Epidemiologia e Serviços de Saúde. 2007;16(1):19-31.

25. Brazil. National Traffic Department (DENATRAN). Statistical Bulletin. Seguradora Líder DPVAT. Brasília; 2014. v.4.

26. Sothmann J, Stander J, Kruger N, Dunn R. Epidemiology of acute spinal cord injuries in the Groote Schuur Hospital Acute Spinal Cord Injury (GSH ASCI) Unit, Cape Town, South Africa, over the past 11 years. S Afr Med J. 2015; 105(10):835-9.

27. Soares A, Santos NR. Financing the Unified Health System in the FHC, Lula and Dilma governments. Saúde Debate 2014;38(100): 18-25.

28. Marinho MGS, Cesse EAP, Bezerra AFB, Sousa IMC, Fontbonne A, Carvalho EF. Cost analysis of health care for patients with diabetes mellitus and hypertension in a public health unit of reference in Recife - Brazil. Arq Bras Endocrinol Metab. 2011 ;55(6):406-11.

29. Brazil. Ministry of Labour and Employment. Brazilian Classification of Occupations. Brasilia; 2002.

30. Brazilian Institute of Geography and Statistics. Territorial Units of the Geographic Mesoregion Level. Rio de Janeiro: IBGE, 2000.

31. Mello LR, Espíndola G; Silva FM, Bernardes CL Spinal cord injury. Prospective study of 92 cases. Arq Bras Neurocir. 2004;23(4):151-6.

32. Scopel G, Jacob Júnior C, Brazolino MAN, Cardoso IM, Batista Júnior JL, Sogame LC, et al. Evaluation of the epidemiological profile of traumatic spinal cord injury in a spine service in the state of Espírito Santo. Arq Bras Neurocir. 2016;35(1): in press.

33. Anderle DV, Joaquim AF, Soares MS, Miura FK, Silva FL, Veiga JCE, et al. Epidemiological evaluation of patients with spinal cord injury operated on at the Professor Carlos da Silva Lacaz State Hospital. Coluna/Columna. 2010;9(1):58-61.

34. Tavares CB, Sousa EB, Borges IBC, Godinho Júnior AA, Freire Neto NG. Epidemiological profile of patients with thoracic and lumbar fractures treated surgically at the Neurosurgery Service of the Hospital de Base do Distrito Federal (Brasília-Brazil). Arq Bras Neurocir. 2013;32(1): 19-25.

35. Souza ER. Masculinity and violence in Brazil: contributions to reflection in the field of health. Ciênc Saúde Coletiva. 2005; 10(1):59-70.

36. Rodrigues LCL, Bortoletto A, Matsumoto MH. Epidemiology of surgical thoracolumbar fractures in eastern São Paulo. Coluna/Columna. 2010;9(2):132-7.

37. Morais DF. Traumatic spinal cord injury: epidemiological, clinical and radiological aspects [PhD Thesis]. São José do Rio Preto (SP): São José do Rio Preto Medical School; 2013.

38. Chamberlain JD, Deriaz O, Hund-Georgiadis M, Meier S, Anke Scheel- Sailer A, Schubert M, et al. Epidemiology and contemporary risk profile of traumatic spinal cord injury in Switzerland. Inj Epidemiol. 2015;2(1):28-39.

39. Custódio NRO, Carneiro MR, Feres CC, Lima GHS, Jubé MRR, Watanabe LE, et al. Spinal cord injury at the Centro de Reabilitação e Readaptação Dr. Henrique Santillo (CRER-GO). Coluna/Columna. 2009;8(3):265-8.

40. Wu JC, Chen YC, Liu L, Chen TJ, Huang WC, Cheng H, et al. Effects of age, gender, and socio-economic status on the incidence of spinal cord injury: an assessment using the eleven-

year comprehensive nationwide database of Taiwan. J Neurotrauma. 2012; 29(5):889-97.

41. World Health Organisation. International Perspectives on Spinal Cord Injury. Malta: WHO; 2013. 250p.

42. Morais DF, Spotti AR, Cohen MI, Mussi SE, Melo Neto JS, Tognola WA. Epidemiological profile of patients with spinal cord injury treated at a tertiary hospital. Coluna/Columna. 2013; 12(2): 149-52.

43. Jácomo AAE, Garcia ACF. Analysis of motorbike accidents at the Centro de Reabilitação e Readaptação Dr. Henrique Santillo (CRER). Acta Fisiatr. 2011;18(3):124-9.

44. Hasler RM, Exadaktylos AK, Bouamra O, Benneker LM, Clancy M, Sieber R, et al. Epidemiology and predictors of spinal injury in adult major trauma patients: European cohort study. Eur Spine J. 2011 ;20(12):2174-80.

45. Guzelkucuk U, Demir Y, Kesikburun S, Yasar E, Yilmaz B. Spinal cord injury in older population in Turkey. Spinal Cord. 2014;52(11):850-4.

46. Blanes L, Lourenço L, Carmagnani MIS, Ferreira LM. Clinicai and socio- demographic characteristics of persons with traumatic paraplegia living in São Paulo, BraziL Arq Neuropsiquiatr. 2009;67(2b):388-90.

47. Santiago LMDM, Barbosa LCDS, Guerra RO, Melo FRLV. Sociodemographic and clinical aspects of men with traumatic spinal cord injury in an urban centre in northeastern Brazil. Arq Bras Ciênc Saúde. 2012;37(3):137- 42.

48. DeVivo MJ. Epidemiology of traumatic spinal cord injury: trends and future implications. Spinal Cord. 2012;50(5):365-72.

49. Rahimi-Movaghar V, Sayyah MK, Akbari H, Khorramirouz R, Rasouli MR, Moradi-Lakeh M, et al. Epidemiology of traumatic spinal cord injury in developing countries: a systematic review. Neuroepidemiology. 2013;41(2):65- 85.

50. Barras MN, Basso RC. Spinal cord trauma - epidemiological profile of patients treated by the public service in the state of Goiás between 2000 and 2003. Fisioter Bras. 2005;6(2):141-4.

51. National Institute of Science and Technology. Evolution of the car and motorbike fleet in Brazil: 2001-2012 (Report 2013). Rio de Janeiro: INCT, 2013.

52. Bertoncello KCG, Cavalcanti CDK, Ilha P. Analysis of the patient profile as a victim of multiple traumas. Cogitara Enferm. 2012;17(4):717-23.

53. Oliveira TAB, Andrade SMS, Prado GO, Fernandes RB, Gusmão MS, Gomes EGF, et al. Epidemiology of spine fractures in motorbike accident victims. Coluna/Columna. 2016;15(1):65-7.

54. Waiselfisz JJ. Map of violence 2013: road traffic and motorbike accidents

Rio de Janeiro: CEBELA, 2013.

55. Bachieri G, Barras AJD. Traffic accidents in Brazil from 1998 to 2010: many changes and few results. Rev Saúde Pública. 2011 ;45(5):949-56.

56. Fava JE. Traumatic spinal cord injury: clinical and epidemiological characteristics of patients treated at a highly complex hospital in Campo Grande/Mato Grosso do Sul [Dissertation]. Campo Grande (MS): Federal University of Mato Grosso do Sul; 2011.

57. Tugcu I, Tok F, Yilmaz B, Gõktepe AS, Alaca R, Yaziciog6lu K, et al. Epidemiologic data of the patients with spinal cord injury: seven years' experience of a single centre. Ulus Travma Acil Cerrahi Derg. 2011 ;17(6):533-8.

58. Carvalho ICCM, Saraiva IS. Profile of trauma victims treated by the mobile emergency care service. R Interd. 2015;8(1): 137-48.

59. Pimentel MG, Gomes EGF, Gusmão MS, De Amorim Júnior DC, Simões MTV, Gomes JF, et al. Epidemiological study of spinal cord trauma caused by firearm projectiles at the Bahia State General Hospital. Coluna/Columna. 2012;11 (4):298-301.

60. Touno VL. Spinal trauma in Brazil: an analysis of hospital admissions [Dissertation]. São Paulo (SP): University of São Paulo; 2008.

61. Karimi M. The effects of orthosis on thoracolumbar fracture healing: a review of the literature. J Orthop. 2015;12(2):230-7.

62. Fernandes RB, Gomes EGF, Gusmão MS, Amorim Júnior DC, Simões MTV, Gomes JF, et al. Clinical epidemiological study of spinal fractures. Coluna/Columna. 2012;11(3):230-3.

63. Bernardi DM. Epidemiological profile of surgery for spinomedullary injury at a referral hospital in a country town of Brazil. Coluna/Columna. 2014; 13(2): 136-8.

64. Wyndaele M, Wyndaele J-J. Incidence, prevalence and epidemiology of spinal cord injury: what learns a worldwide literature survey? Spinal Cord. 2006;44:523-9.

65. Lenehan B, Street J, Kwon BK, Noonan V, Zhang H, Fisher CG, et al. The Epidemiology of traumatic spinal cord injury in British Columbia, Canada. Spine. 2012;37(4):321-9.

66. Yang R, Guo L, Wang P, Huang L, Tang Y, Wang W, et al. Epidemiology of spinal cord injuries and risk factors for complete injuries in Guangdong, China: a retrospective study. PLoS One. 2014;9(1): 1-10.

67. Macciocchi S, Seel RT, Warshowsky A, Thompson N, Barlow K. Co-occurring traumatic brain injury and acute spinal cord injury rehabilitation outcomes. Arch Phys Med Rehabil. 2012;93:1788-94.

68. Kumar I, Chaudhuri A, Acharya S, Ghosh PK, Acharya PP, De A. Recovery patterns of spinal cord injury after traumatic cervical cord injury in a developing country. Saudi J Sports Med. 2016; 16(2): 128-32.

69. Sousa EPD, Araújo OF, Sousa CLM, Muniz MV, Oliveira IR, Freire Neto NG. Main complications of spinal cord injury in patients admitted to the neurosurgery unit of the Base Hospital of the Federal District. Commun. Ciênc Saúde. 2013; 24(4):321-330.

70. Kucukdurmaz F, Alijanipour P. Current concepts in orthopedic management of multiple trauma. Open Orthop J. 2015;9(1):275-82.

71. Santos EAS, Santos Filho WJ, Possatti LL, Bittencourt LRA, Fontoura EAF, Botelho RV. Clinical complications in patients with severe cervical spinal trauma: a ten-year prospective study. Arq Neuropsiquiatr. 2012;70(7):524-8.

72. Grossman RG, Frankowski RF, Burau KD, Toups EG, Crommett JW, Johnson MM, et al. Incidence and severity of acute complications after spinal cord injury. J Neurosurg Spine. 2012; 17(1): 119-28.

73. Lindgren M, Unosson M, Fredrikson M, Ek AC. Immobility - a major risk factor for development of pressure ulcers among adult hospitalised patients: a prospective study. Scand J Caring Sei. 2004;18:57-64.

74. Chopra T, Marchaim D, Awali RA, Levine M, Sathyaprakash S, Chalana IK, et al. Risk factors and acute in-hospital costs for infected pressure ulcers among gunshot-spinal cord injury victims in southeastern Michigan. Am J Infect Contrai. 2016;44(3):315-9.

75. Scheel-Sailer A, Wyss A, Boldt C, Post MW, Lay V. Prevalence, location, grade of pressure ulcers and association with specific patient characteristics in adult spinal cord injury patients during the hospital stay: a prospective cohort study. Spinal Cord. 2013;51(11):828-33.

76. Sekulic A, Nikolic AK, Bukumiric Z, Trajkovic G, Corac A, Jankovic S Analysis of the factors influencing development of urinary tract infection in patients with spinal cord injuries. Vojnosanit Pregl. 2015;72(12): 1074-9.

77. Stephan K, Huber S, Hãberle S, Kanz KG, Búhren V, Van Griensven M, et al. Spinal cord injury--incidence, prognosis, and outcome: an analysis of the TraumaRegister DGU. Spine J. 2015; 15(9): 1994-2001.

78. Morais DF, Melo Neto JS, Spotti AR, Tognola WA. Predictors of clinical complications in patients with spinal cord trauma. Coluna/Columna. 2014; 13(2): 139-42.

79. Bliemel C, Lefering R, Buecking B, Frink M, Struewer J, Krueger A, et al. Early or delayed stabilisation in severely injured patients with spinal fractures? Current surgical objectivity according to the Trauma Registry of DGU: treatment of spine injuries in polytrauma patients. J Trauma Acute Gare Surg. 2014;76(2):366-73.

80. Bourassa-Moreau É, Mac-Thiong JM, Ehrmann Feldman D, Thompson C, Parent S. Complications in acute phase hospitalisation of traumatic spinal cord injury: does surgical timing matter? J Trauma Acute Gare Surg. 2013 Mar;74(3):849-54.

81. Musienko P, Heutschi J, Friedli L, Van Den Brand R, Courtine G. Multi- system neurorehabilitative strategies to restore motor functions following severe spinal cord injury. Exp NeuroL 2012;235(1): 100-9.
82. Boland RA, Lin CSY, Engel S, Kiernan MC. Adaptation of motor function after spinal cord injury: novel insights into spinal shock. Brain. 2011;134(2):495- 505.
83. Galea MP, Dunlop SA, Marshall R, Clark J, Churilov L. Early exercise after spinal cord injury ('Switch-On'): study protocol for a randomised controlled trial. Trials. 2015; 16:7.
84. Armada-da-Silva PA, Pereira C, Amado S, Veloso AP. Role of physical exercise for improving posttraumatic nerve regeneration. Int Rev Neurobiol. 2013;109:125-49.
85. Fakhoury M. Spinal cord injury: overview of experimental approaches used to restore locomotor activity. Rev Neurosci. 2015;26(4):397-405.
86. Hubli M, Dietz V. The physiological basis of neurorehabilitation - locomotor training after spinal cord injury. J Neuroeng Rehabil. 2013;10:5.
87. Horn SD, Smout RJ, DeJong G, Dijkers MP, Hsieh CH, Lammertse D, et al. Association of various comorbidity measures with spinal cord injury rehabilitation outcomes. Arch Phys Med Rehab 2013;94(4):75-86.
88. Crane DA, Hoffman JM, Reyes MR. Benefits of an exercise wellness programme after spinal cord injury. J Spinal Cord Med. 2015;25:1-5.
89. Sharma H, Alilain WA, Sadhu A, Silver J. Treatments to restore respiratory function after spinal cord injury and their implications for regeneration, plasticity and adaptation. Exp NeuroL 2012;235(1):18-25.
90. Ferreira LL, Marino LHC, Cavenaghi S. Physiotherapeutic Action in Spinal Cord Injury in the Intensive Care Unit: literature update. Rev Neurocienc. 2012;20(4):612-7.
91. Postma K, Vlemmix LY, Haisma JA, de Groot S, Sluis TA, Stam HJ, et al. Longitudinal association between respiratory muscle strength and cough capacity in persons with spinal cord injury: An explorative analysis of data from a randomised controlled trial. J Rehabil Med. 2015;47(8):722-6.
92. Pelletier CA, Latimer-Cheung AE, Warburton DE, Hicks AL. Direct referral and physical activity counselling upon discharge from spinal cord injury rehabilitation. Spinal Cord. 2014;52(5):392-5.
93. Ray AD, Udhoji S, Mashtare TL, Fisher NM. A combined inspiratory and expiratory muscle training program improves respiratory muscle strength and fatigue in multiple sclerosis. Arch Phys Med Rehabil. 2013;94(10): 1964-70.
94. Scivoletto G, Morgant B, Molinar M. Early versus delayed inpatient spinal cord injury

rehabilitation: an Italian study. Arch Phys Med Rehabil. 2005;86:512- 6.

95. Wuermser LA, Ho CH, Chiodo AE, Priebe MM, Kirshblum SC, Scelza WM. Spinal Cord Injury Medicine. 2. Acute Care Management of Traumatic and Nontraumatic Injury. Arch Phys Med Rehabil. 2007;88(1):55-61.

96. Andresen SR, Biering-Sorensen F, Hagen EM,Nielsen JF, Bach FW, Finnerup NB. Pain, spasticity and quality of life in individuals with traumatic spinal cord injury in Denmark. Spinal Cord. 2016: in press.

97. Campos AB, Gonçalves RC, Carvalho CRF. Doctors' assessment of the referral of patients with neurological dysfunctions for physiotherapy care. Fisioter Pesqui. 2006;13(3):36-42.

98. Jorge LL, Sugawara AT, Carneiro MSO. Patients admitted to a general hospital referred to Physical Medicine: epidemiological profile and functional level. Acta Fisiatr. 2006; 13(3): 124-9.

99. Sweet S, Noreau L, Leblond J, Dumont F. Understanding quality of life in adults with spinal cord injury via SCI - related needs and secondary complications. Fali. 2014;20(4):321-8.

100. Creôncio SCE, Moura JC, Rangel BLR. Clinical and epidemiological aspects of spinal cord trauma at the Hospital de Urgências e Traumas - Petrolina-PE. J Bras Neurocirurg. 2012;23(3):211-6.

101. Pereira CU, Jesus RM. Epidemiology of spinal cord injury. J Bras Neurocirurg. 2011;22(2):26-31.

102. Hagen EM. How to prevent early mortality due to spinal cord injuries? New evidence & update. Indian J Med Res. 2014;140(1):5-7.

103. Costa RC, Caliri MHL, Costa LS, Gamba MA. Factors associated with the occurrence of pressure ulcers in spinal cord injured patients. Rev Neurocienc. 2013;21(1):60-8.

104. Cardenas DD, Hoffman JM, Kirshblum S, McKinley W. Etiology and incidence of rehospitalisation after traumatic spinal cord injury: a multicenter analysis. Arch Phys Med Rehabil. 2004;85(11):1757-63.

105. Lalwani S, Singh V, Trikha V, Sharma V, Kumar S, Bagla R, et al. Mortality profile of patients with traumatic spinal injuries at a levei I trauma care centre in India. Indian J Med Res. 2014;140:40-5.

106. Neumann CR, Brasil AV, Alberts F. Risk factors for mortality in traumatic cervical spinal cord injury: Brazilian data. J Trauma. 2009;67:67-70.

107. Saunders LL, Selassie AW, Hill EG, Nicholas JS, Varma AK, Lackland DT et al. Traumatic spinal cord injury mortality, 1981-1998. J Trauma. 2009;66(1): 184-90.

108. Chiu WT, Lin HC, Lam C, Chu SF, Chiang YH, Tsai SH. Review paper: epidemiology of traumatic spinal cord injury: comparisons between developed and developing countries. Asia Pac J Public Health. 2010;22(1):9-18.
109. Santos TSC, Guimarães RM, Boeira SF. Epidemiology of spinal cord trauma in public emergencies in the municipality of Rio de Janeiro. Esc Anna Nery. 2012; 16(4)747-53.

Special thanks from the author

To my husband **Juliano Veronezi,** for his unconditional support at all times, especially when I was uncertain. Without you, no achievement would have been worthwhile!

To my parents **Cirilo** and **Marcília,** who worthily introduced me to the importance of family and the path of honesty and persistence.

To my siblings **Daniela, Isabela** and **Thales,** the most dedicated people I know, who exemplify professional ethics and competence exercised with tenderness and humanisation.

To **Prof Dr Yvens Barbosa Fernandes,** my thanks for the opportunity to do this work alongside someone who inspires wisdom and admiration.

Finally, to the teaching and management staff of the **Department of Neurology at the State University of Campinas (UNICAMP),** who provided the window through which I now see a higher horizon.

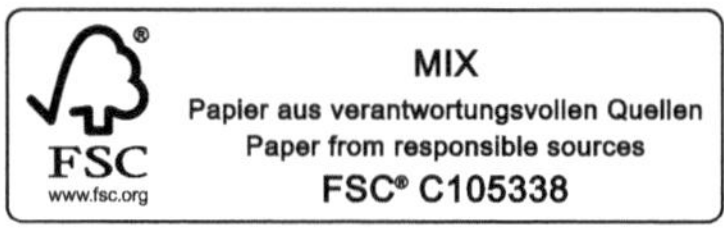

Printed by Books on Demand GmbH, Norderstedt / Germany